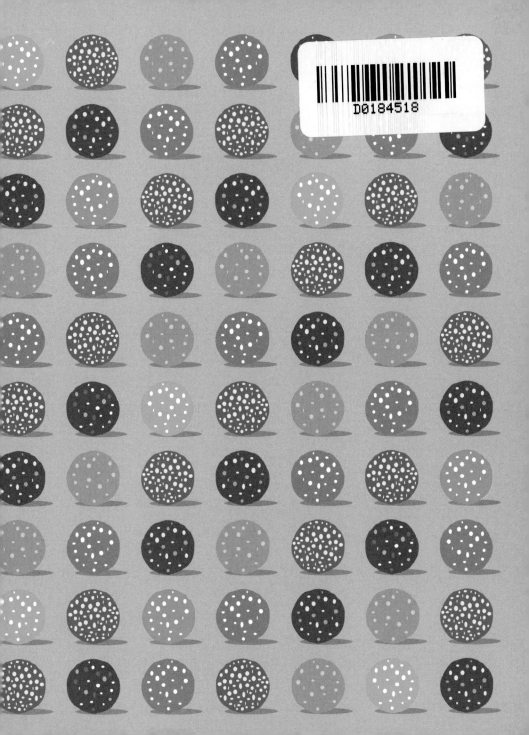

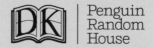

Penguin
Random
House

Writers Kate Turner, with Annie Nichols

Project Designer Sonia Moore

Senior Art Editor Alison Gardner

Jacket Designer Nicola Powling

Jacket Editor Francesca Young

Pre-production Producer Andy Hilliard

Print Producer Stephanie McConnell

Creative Technical Support
Sonia Charbonnier

Photography Will Heap

Managing Editor Lisa Dyer

Managing Art Editor
Marianne Markham

Art Director Maxine Pedliham

Publishing Director Mary-Clare Jerram

First published in Great Britain in 2016

By Dorling Kindersley Limited, 80 Strand, London WC2R 0RL

Copyright © 2016 Dorling Kindersley
A Penguin Random House Company

4 6 8 10 9 7 5 3
006-291546-Jan/16

ISBN: 978-0-2412-4997-0

Printed and bound in Slovakia

**Discover more at
www.dk.com**

ENERGY Bites

*High-protein recipes for
increased vitality & wellness*

CONTENTS

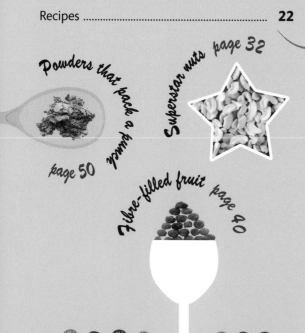

Powders that pack a punch page 50

Superstar nuts page 32

Fibre-filled fruit page 40

PICK A RECIPE

Treat yourself to a power-packed snack with 7 savoury and 8 sweet, simple-to-make superball recipes.

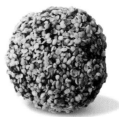

HEMP-COATED
QUINOA CRUNCHERS
Page 30

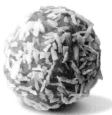

TROPICAL
IMMUNE BOOSTERS
Page 42

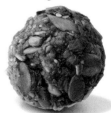

SUPERFOOD
GRANOLA BALLS
Page 52

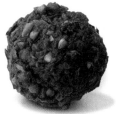

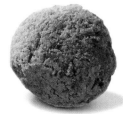

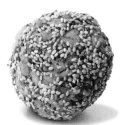

CARROT & BEETROOT
BUCKWHEAT BALLS
Page 24

PEA GREEN
HIGH-PROTEIN MUNCHERS
Page 26

NUT & SEED
NUTRIENT BOOSTERS
Page 28

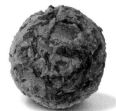

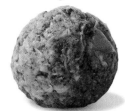

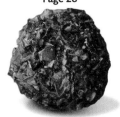

SWEET POTATO
CHILLI BITES
Page 34

BROCCOLI & MACA
POWERHOUSE BALLS
Page 36

KALE-COVERED
COCONUT BLASTS
Page 38

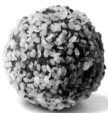

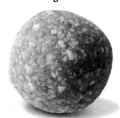

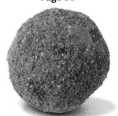

PEANUT BUTTER
& BANANA BALLS
Page 44

APPLE "PIE"
ANTIOXIDANT BITES
Page 46

FRUIT & NUT
BUILD-A-BALLS
Page 48

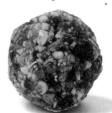

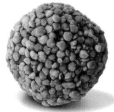

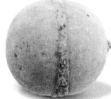

CRANBERRY & FIG
SPICE BITES
Page 54

RAW CHOCOLATE
INSTANT ENERGY TREATS
Page 56

AVOCADO & BANANA
RECOVERY ICE BITES
Page 58

SO HERE'S WHY THEY'RE **AWESOME...**

Eating deliciously healthy, all-natural food is becoming a top priority for more and more people, especially if you lead a busy life or have a growing family to feed. We all want tasty meals and snacks that will make us feel amazing and are quick and easy to prepare. That's where Energy Bites come in! All of the recipes in this book are vegetarian, gluten- and dairy-free, energy-packed, and protein-rich; some are "raw" and all of them are free of refined sugars. So what makes them so good for you? These recipes are created with health benefits in mind, and each one should pack a serious nutrient power punch and deliver a host of vitamins, minerals and phytochemicals (such as antioxidants and anti-inflammatories) that help support and protect the working systems of your body.

The bites are ball-shaped, loaded with goodness, and easy to grab for breakfast, lunch, dinner, or as a tasty treat. They're portable nuggets of intense nutrition and are handy for adding to kids' lunchboxes, taking to the office, enjoying on a picnic, or even simply as a little taste of decadence, knowing that all of the recipes are incredibly good for

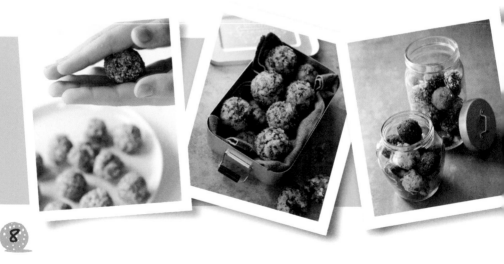

you. Every bite is full of "superfood" ingredients, so you can expect a completely natural health boost and an awesome sense of wellbeing from these vitality-packed goodies. You don't get much better than that!

Mix and match

The 15 recipes in this book are all fabulous in their own right, but feel free to experiment with your favourite flavours. The basic "Energy Bite formula" is given on page 16, and over the next few pages there are plenty of ideas for ingredients to incorporate in your own creations. Whether you're looking for a pre-workout stamina boost, a muscle-building protein hit, support for your immune system, or even a cool iced treat to help you rehydrate, there's an Energy Bite for you!

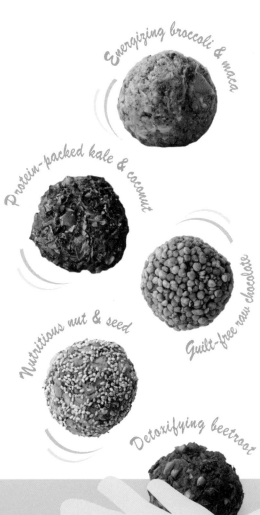

Energizing broccoli & maca

Protein-packed kale & coconut

Guilt-free raw chocolate

Nutritious nut & seed

Detoxifying beetroot

" *Make mine a* **cranberry & fig** *to go please!*"

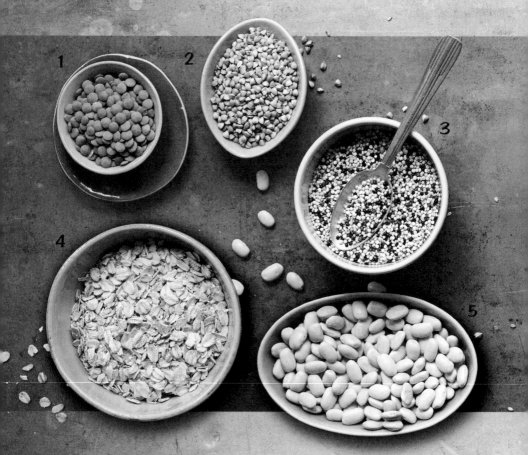

20 **TOP INGREDIENTS**

1 Lentils A great source of plant protein, lentils are also high in fibre, magnesium, potassium, and folate (vitamin B9).

2 Buckwheat Gluten-free buckwheat has high amounts of vitamins, minerals, and fibre, and keeps the body fuelled with slow-release energy.

3 Quinoa Containing all the essential amino acids that our bodies need, quinoa is loaded with manganese, magnesium, and phosphorus, vital for wellbeing.

4 Oats One of the best sources of soluble fibre, oats help to lower cholesterol, and leave you feeling energized for hours.

5 Beans High in protein, when combined with a grain, such as brown rice, beans provide a complete plant-protein source on a par with meat!

6 Sesame seeds Full of vitamins, minerals, and phytosterols that support the immune system, sesame seeds also help regulate

The **20 ingredients** featured below and on the following pages come top of the list for Energy Bite recipes – they are all incredibly good for you and pack a **serious superfood punch**! For the best possible results, buy (or, better still, grow) **organic ingredients** whenever possible.

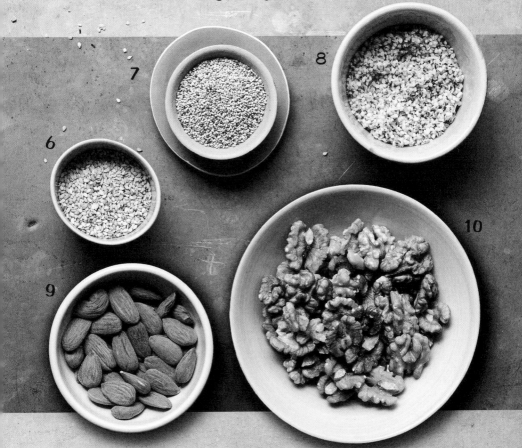

blood cholesterol and may even help to fight cancer!

7 Chia seeds These tiny seeds contain high levels of omega-3 fatty acids and have five times more calcium than cows' milk. They are rich in antioxidants, anti-inflammatories, and energy-enhancing fibre.

8 Hemp seeds This source of vegetarian protein helps to regulate energy levels. Hemp seeds are also packed with zinc, magnesium, and calcium, and are a powerful anti-inflammatory.

9 Almonds Loaded with more vitamin E than any other nut, plus bone-friendly calcium,

versatile almonds can be flaked, ground, left whole, and even made into milk.

10 Walnuts Packing a massive protein punch, walnuts are particularly high in cholesterol-lowering compounds, as well as the stress-busting hormone melatonin.

"These ingredients are crammed with goodness!"

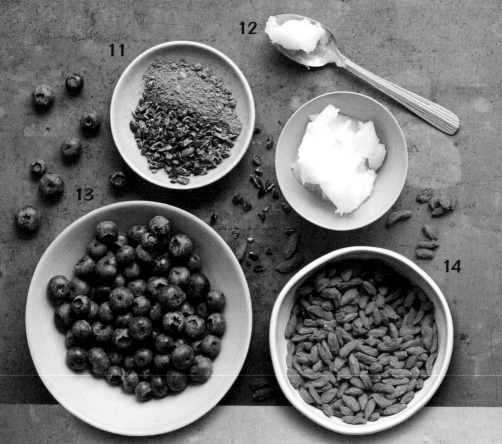

11

12

13

14

11 Cacao Chocolate in its most natural form. Packed with antioxidants and vitamins, it is said to enhance motivation and feelings of pleasure!

12 Coconut oil With potent antibacterial, antifungal, and antimicrobial properties, coconut oil is also the richest natural source of lauric acid, which is said to boost immunity and fight disease.

13 Blueberries Filled with antioxidants, fibre, vitamin C, and cancer-fighting compounds, blueberries are said to be good for the heart, and even to help improve eyesight and memory.

14 Goji berries Containing more beta-carotene than any other plant, goji berries also have more iron, gram for gram, than steak!

15 Avocado Full of antioxidants, avocados are also high in healthy fats, fibre, potassium, vitamin E, and magnesium. They are amazing for the skin.

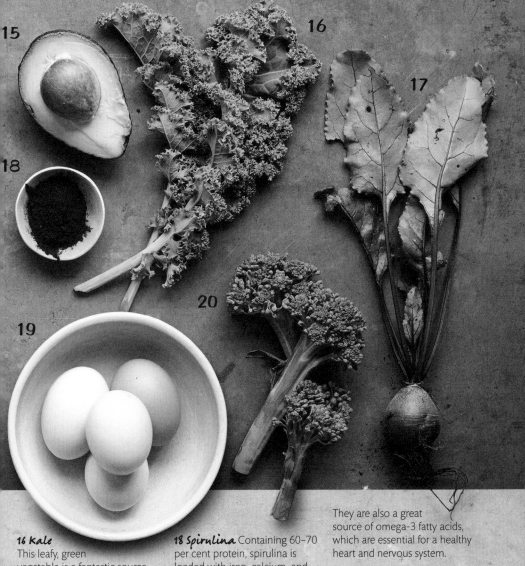

16 Kale
This leafy, green vegetable is a fantastic source of antioxidants, protein, iron, fibre, and calcium.

17 Beetroot Known to lower blood pressure and thought to be a potent detoxifier, beetroot also supports heart health.

18 Spirulina Containing 60–70 per cent protein, spirulina is loaded with iron, calcium, and vitamins, is great for healthy skin, and supports the nervous system.

19 Eggs High in protein, with 20 amino acids in a super-digestible form, eggs provide us with every single vitamin except vitamin C.

They are also a great source of omega-3 fatty acids, which are essential for a healthy heart and nervous system.

20 Broccoli One of the most protein-rich vegetables, broccoli is also packed with vitamins and antioxidants, plus compounds that fight illness, improve reproductive health, and reduce the risk of heart disease.

13

Other Great INGREDIENTS

Nuts & seeds

Brazils A fantastic source of monounsaturated fatty acids and selenium, Brazil nuts are great for the hair and skin.

Cashews An abundant source of essential minerals such as manganese, potassium, iron, magnesium, and zinc.

Golden linseed (flaxseed) One of the best plant-based sources of omega-3 fatty acids around, and a great source of B vitamins.

Hazelnuts Incredibly nutritious, hazelnuts have high levels of dietary fibre and folate, an important B-complex vitamin.

Pecans A source of antioxidant ellagic acid, which can help protect the body from disease.

Pistachios A fantastic source of healthy fats, protein, and copper, vital for red blood cell production.

Pumpkin seeds A source of tryptophan, which is converted by the body into sleep-regulating neurotransmitter serotonin.

Sunflower seeds Packed full of essential amino acids, and a rich source of folic acid.

Fruit & vegetables

Apples Dried or fresh, apples add sweetness to recipes while delivering C and B vitamins and fibre.

Apricots An excellent source of vitamin A, essential for eye health, and heart-healthy potassium.

Banana Rich in potassium and easy to digest – bananas are great for instant energy.

Carrot Exceptionally high in vitamin A and beta-carotene, one of the most powerful natural antioxidants.

Celery An excellent source of dietary fibre and vitamin K, celery also supports eye health.

Chillies Capsaicin, which gives chillies their heat, has antibacterial and cancer-fighting properties. They are also very high in vitamin C.

Coconut Contains lauric acid, which increases levels of "good" HDL cholesterol in the blood.

Edamame (soya) beans Usually sold podded and frozen, these beans are an excellent source of protein, iron, and fibre.

Figs An excellent source of antioxidants, plus chlorogenic acid, which can help to balance blood sugar levels.

Garlic Contains allicin, which has been found to have antibacterial, antifungal, and antiviral properties.

Ginger Contains the essential oil gingerol, with anti-inflammatory and painkilling properties. Can also help to reduce nausea.

Mangoes High in amino acids and A and B vitamins, the fruit can be used fresh or dried. It has antioxidant compounds that are thought to protect against cancer.

Onions Rich in chromium, a trace mineral that helps the body regulate insulin production.

Orange/lemon/lime Excellent sources of vitamin C, plus citric acid that can aid digestion.

Peas Rich in phyto-nutrients, vitamin C, and folate. Frozen peas are just as high in vitamins as fresh.

Raisins A great source of sweetness and energy, raisins also have several times more fibre than fresh grapes.

Red pepper Contains concentrated levels of vitamin C, plus vitamin A, and essential B vitamins.

Seaweed Nutrient-dense, low-calorie seaweed is a potent source of iodine, important for thyroid function.

Sweet potato These versatile vegetables are a much richer source of fibre, antioxidants, and vitamins than ordinary potatoes.

Tomato Contains lycopene, a powerful antioxidant that may help to protect against cancer, as well as choline, an important nutrient that helps with sleep, muscle movement, and memory.

Grains & pulses

Brown rice Wholegrains like brown rice can help reduce the risk of heart disease. Brown rice is also rich in selenium and manganese.

Bulgur wheat Containing iron and B vitamins, bulgur wheat is a great source of energy, fibre, and protein, though it is not gluten free.

Chickpeas (incl. gram flour) Including high levels of iron, vitamin B6, magnesium, and fibre, chickpeas are also a fantastic vegetarian source of protein.

Yellow split peas Extremely beneficial for health, split peas contain soluble fibre to help lower cholesterol and regulate blood sugar, and cancer-fighting isoflavones.

The sticky stuff

Apple cider vinegar An ancient folk remedy, apple cider vinegar has insulin-regulating properties, helping to lower blood sugar levels.

Coconut milk Nutritious and dairy-free, coconut milk offers all the health benefits of coconut while adding a rich flavour to recipes.

Maple syrup Pure maple syrup has a unique sweet flavour, contains immune-boosting zinc, and also has antioxidant properties.

Miso paste Made from fermented soya beans, Japanese miso paste is high in complete proteins that contain all of the body's essential amino acids.

Olive oil Rich in monounsaturated fatty acids, renowned for their cholesterol-balancing properties.

Rice syrup An alternative to refined sugar, rice syrup offers many of the B vitamins and minerals that are found in brown rice.

Tahini (crushed sesame seeds) This creamy paste is a fantastic source of calcium, potassium, lecithin, magnesium, and iron.

Tamari A wheat-free soy sauce, tamari provides niacin (vitamin B3), manganese, and the mood-enhancing amino acid, tryptophan.

Raw honey With antibacterial, antifungal, and antiviral properties, raw honey is also a powerful natural antioxidant and healer.

Vegetable stock Used in the hemp-coated quinoa crunchers recipe on page 30, this is easy to make – just fry onions in a large pan with a little oil, add vegetables such as celery, garlic, mushrooms and carrots, and herbs such as thyme, bay and rosemary, top up with plenty of water and simmer for 40 minutes, then strain and store in the fridge for up to a week, or the freezer for up to three months.

Spices

Allspice Also known as Jamaican pepper, allspice has a warming flavour and anti-inflammatory properties. It contains the essential oil eugenol, which is antiseptic.

Cinnamon Contains the highest antioxidant strength of all natural foods, and is also an excellent source of essential minerals.

Cloves High in eugenol, an essential oil with local anaesthetic and antiseptic properties.

Cumin These distinctively-flavoured seeds are an excellent source of health-benefiting essential oils.

Garam masala A blend of several spices commonly used in Indian cookery, such as coriander seeds, cumin, cardamom, mustard seeds, fenugreek, and caraway.

Nutmeg Best freshly ground or grated, nutmeg may have antifungal, antidepressant, and antioxidant properties.

Paprika Made by grinding dried capsicum peppers to a powder, paprika can be hot, sweet or smoky, and has antibacterial and anti-inflammatory properties.

Turmeric A powerful anti-inflammatory and immune booster, turmeric has been used for centuries in Chinese and Indian medicine.

Herbs

Basil With exceptionally high levels of antioxidant beta-carotene and vitamin A, basil also contains eye-protecting zeaxanthin.

Coriander A rich source of vitamins K, A, and C, both the leaves and the seeds also have antioxidant properties.

Mint The flavour comes from the essential oil menthol, which has painkilling properties, and it can also aid digestion.

Parsley Rich in antioxidants, parsley is also high in vitamin K, which may help to promote bone health.

Thyme Contains antiseptic thymol and is packed with potassium that can help regulate blood pressure.

The rest

Acai powder Made from dried acai berries, this can boost energy and help support the immune system.

Baobab powder Powdered dried baobab fruit is low in sugar and fat, and rich in vitamin C, calcium, iron, magnesium, and potassium.

Bee pollen Packed with protein, antioxidants, vitamins, and minerals, bee pollen contains nearly all the essential nutrients the body needs.

Lucuma powder The "superfruit" lucuma has been eaten in Peru since 200 AD. Powdered lucuma offers natural sweetness without raising blood sugar, and is also rich in iron.

Maca powder This mineral-rich powder can help to regulate hormones and boost energy, and is even said to improve fertility!

Matcha powder Made from green tea, matcha contains unique, potent antioxidants called catechins, said to have cancer-fighting properties.

Moringa powder Known as the "miracle tree" thanks to its health benefits, moringa leaf is a great source of vitamin A, vitamin C, iron, and calcium.

The Energy Bite FORMULA

There are literally hundreds of ways to combine ingredients to make the perfect "bite". This is just a simple guide to get you started on creating your own versions using basic foodstuffs. The ingredients you choose – *fruit, nuts and seeds, powders*, plus the *sticky stuff* that binds everything together – will depend on what's in your cupboard and what you fancy at the time!

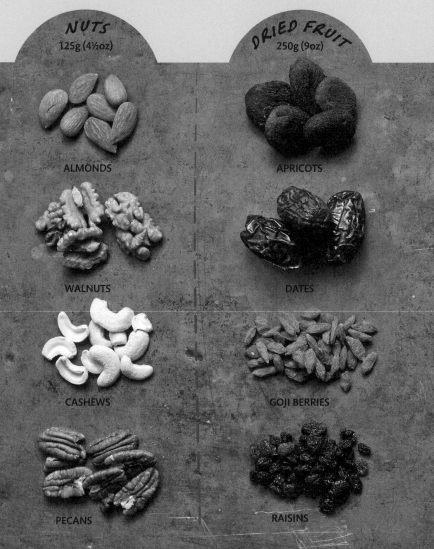

NUTS
125g (4½oz)

DRIED FRUIT
250g (9oz)

ALMONDS

APRICOTS

WALNUTS

DATES

CASHEWS

GOJI BERRIES

PECANS

RAISINS

Simply choose **one ingredient** from **each category** (a combination from the same category is fine, too, as long as you keep to the proportions given – but do omit nuts if you are allergic) and whizz in a food processor. **Shape into balls**, roll in your choice of coating, and firm up in the fridge for 1 hour (if you can wait that long!). Simple.

ta da!

NUTS + DRIED FRUIT + POWDER + STICKY STUFF + COATING =

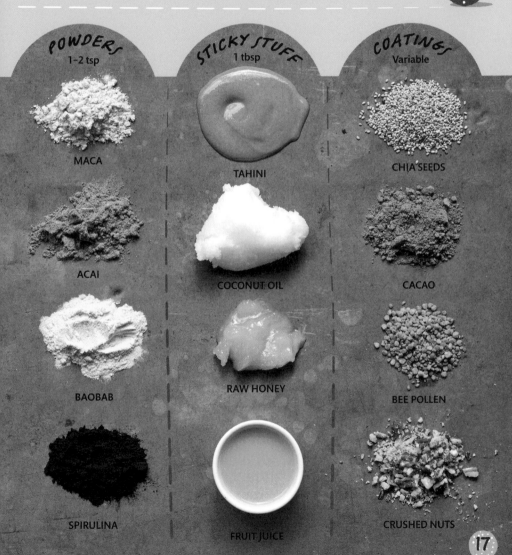

POWDERS
1–2 tsp

MACA

ACAI

BAOBAB

SPIRULINA

STICKY STUFF
1 tbsp

TAHINI

COCONUT OIL

RAW HONEY

FRUIT JUICE

COATINGS
Variable

CHIA SEEDS

CACAO

BEE POLLEN

CRUSHED NUTS

● ● ● ● HOW TO
MAKE NO-BAKES

Apart from being incredibly good for you,
the best thing about **RAW Energy Bites**
is that they are really **EASY** to make.

make the balls about

40mm

in diameter

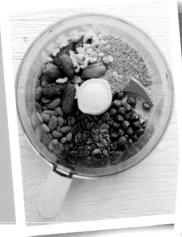

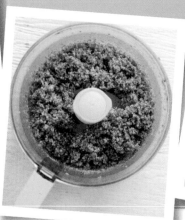

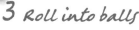

1 start with a food processor

Place all the raw ingredients together in the bowl of a food processor.

2 Form a stiff paste

Whizz the ingredients until they bind together. Depending on the size and power of your processor, you may need to stop it occasionally and push the ingredients down with a spatula before starting it up again.

3 Roll into balls

Divide the mixture into 16 evenly sized portions on a tray or plate. Using your hands, roll the portions into round balls. It will help to have slightly wet hands if the mixture is very sticky.

18

Making by hand

You can still make these Energy Bites without a food processor. Typically, you will need a sharp knife to chop up any dried fruit and herbs, and a pestle and mortar to grind nuts and seeds. You will also need to mash/purée any cooked vegetables with either a mashing utensil or a hand blender. All the ingredients can then be combined in a large bowl.

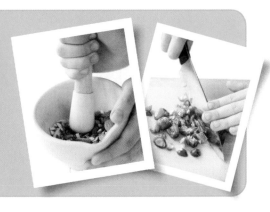

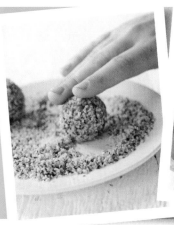

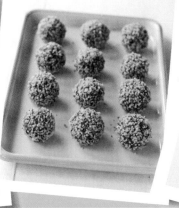

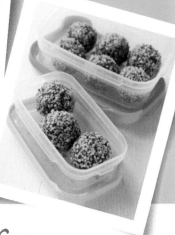

4 Cover in coatings

Spread your choice of coatings evenly on separate plates or trays. Take one of the bites in your hand and roll it gently in the coating. Place on a clean plate.

5 Let them set

Place the bites in the fridge for about an hour before eating to help them keep their shape.

6 Store

If you don't want to eat the bites straightaway, store them in airtight glass or plastic containers in the fridge, where they will last for about a week. They will last for up to a month in the freezer.

HOW TO MAKE **SAVOURY BITES**

SAVOURY bites are slightly more complicated to make, because you may need to STEAM or ROAST some vegetables, or FRY some onions and garlic, before processing.

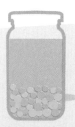

Soak *pulses overnight*

Some of the recipes require soaking dried pulses. Simply place your pulses in a jar, cover with cold water three times their depth, and leave overnight. Drain and rinse under cold running water.

Boil *grains and/or pulses*

Soaked pulses need cooking, as do grains. Place the pulses or grains in a pan and cover with cold water. Bring to the boil, cover, and simmer until soft.

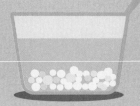

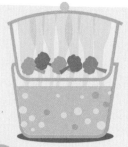

Steam *or roast vegetables*

Some of the recipes require steamed vegetables. Place them in a steamer pan and steam for the required time until soft. Others require roasting. Place the vegetables on a baking tray, cover with foil, and roast until soft. Either way, the aim is to cook the vegetables until soft.

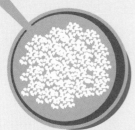

Shallow Fry
vegetables & spices

Most recipes will call for some onion, garlic, and spices to be cooked until soft and translucent. Use a small frying pan on a medium heat with some coconut oil.

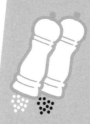

Season

Salt, pepper, and any herbs are added after you've whizzed the main ingredients together in a processor. Use sea salt and freshly ground black pepper for the recipes.

Dividing up the mixture

Savoury mixtures are often quite sticky, and you may find it easier to use a teaspoon to divide the mixture. Place 16 evenly sized, heaped spoonfuls onto a plate or lined baking tray, top each one up with any leftover mixture, and then use your hands to roll into balls. It will help to have slightly wet hands as you roll them.

Bake or shallow-fry?

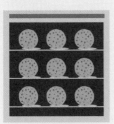

Some of the recipes can be baked in the oven or shallow-fried in coconut oil. So, although there are only 15 recipes in the book, you'll end up with lots of ways to make your bites, all with a different taste. Brilliant!

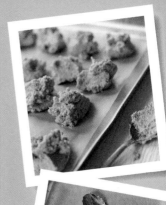

Cool

Leave the balls to cool slightly and harden up on a wire rack before storing them (see page 19).

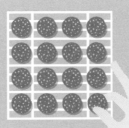

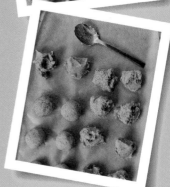

"and now,

15

DELICIOUS,
super-healthy
RECIPES
for **YOU!**"

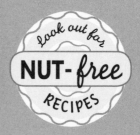

Look out for
NUT-free
RECIPES

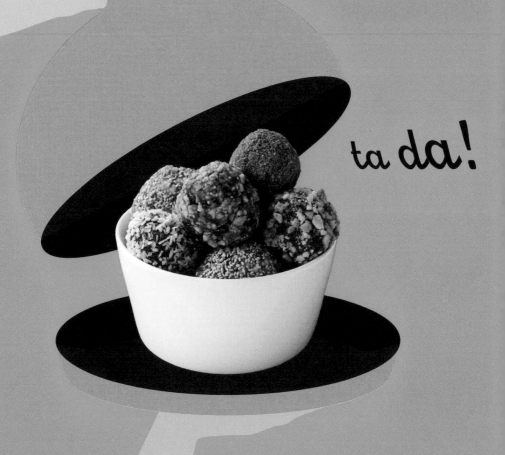

ta da!

CARROT & BEETROOT
BUCKWHEAT BALLS

Includes **BUCKWHEAT** – *an easy-to-digest fruit seed that is* **GLUTEN FREE!**

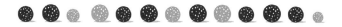

Ingredients

MAKES 16

50g (1¾oz) dried cannellini beans or 45g (1½oz) dried butter beans, soaked overnight (cooked weight about 100g/3½oz)

100g (3½oz) buckwheat groats

175g (6oz) raw beetroot, unpeeled and roughly chopped

175g (6oz) carrots, unpeeled and roughly chopped

50g (1¾oz) Brazil nuts

2 tbsp shelled hemp seeds

4 garlic cloves, crushed

2 tbsp coconut oil

2 tbsp apple cider vinegar

4 tbsp chopped parsley

Method

1 Drain the soaked cannellini beans and rinse under cold running water. Place in a pan with 300ml (10fl oz) boiling water, bring back to the boil, cover, and simmer for 20 minutes until soft. Drain and set aside. If using dried butter beans, simmer for 40–60 minutes until soft.

2 Preheat the oven to 200°C (180°C fan/400°F/Gas 6).

3 Rinse the buckwheat under cold running water. Place in a pan with 300ml (10fl oz) boiling water. Bring back to the boil, cover, and simmer for 10 minutes until soft, but not soggy. Drain and set aside.

4 Steam the beetroot and carrots for 15–20 minutes until soft.

5 Place the remaining ingredients (except the parsley) in a food processor and whizz into a purée. Scrape the mixture into a bowl.

6 Divide it into two. Place half back in the food processor with the carrots and whizz into a purée. Scrape into a clean bowl and set aside.

7 Put the beetroot and remaining mixture in the food processor and whizz into a purée. Scrape into another bowl and set aside.

8 Divide the buckwheat and parsley between the bowls, season both mixtures with salt and pepper, and stir gently until sticky and colourful!

9 Line a large baking tray with parchment paper. Divide the mixture into 16 evenly sized portions and roll into balls.

10 Bake for 20 minutes. Leave to cool for a few minutes on a wire rack before serving hot, or serve them cold.

For one ball: Calories 81 · **Fat** 4.2g · **Carbohydrates** 8.8g · **Sugar** 1.8g
Sodium 11mg · **Fibre** 1.7g · **Protein** 2.3g · **Cholesterol** 0mg

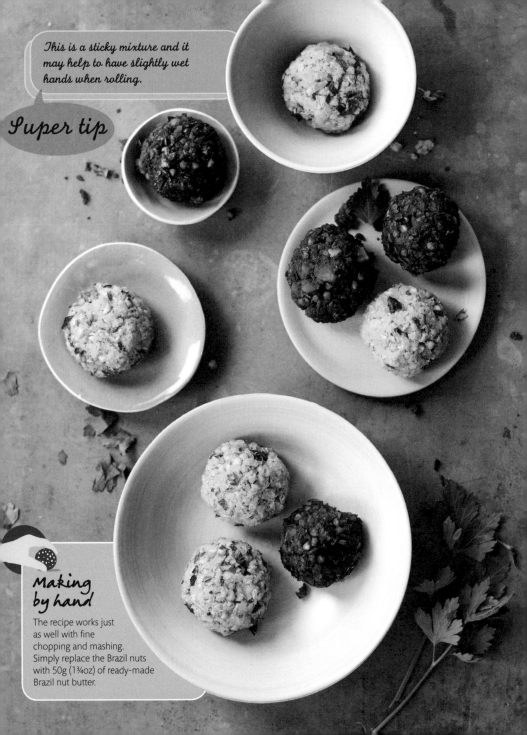

This is a sticky mixture and it may help to have slightly wet hands when rolling.

Super tip

Making by hand

The recipe works just as well with fine chopping and mashing. Simply replace the Brazil nuts with 50g (1¾oz) of ready-made Brazil nut butter.

PEA GREEN
HIGH-PROTEIN MUNCHERS

EDAMAME's high protein and AMINO ACIDS make it great for vegetarians.

Ingredients

MAKES 16

175g (6oz) fresh or frozen podded peas

175g (6oz) frozen podded edamame (soya) beans

50g (1¾oz) rolled oats

3 tbsp peanut, almond, or cashew nut butter

3 tbsp shelled hemp seeds

2 tsp matcha powder (optional)

juice of 1 lemon

2–3 tbsp coconut oil, if frying

Method

1 Blanch the peas and beans in lightly salted water, until just tender, then drain and leave to cool.

2 When they have cooled a little but are still warm, tip the drained peas and beans into the bowl of a food processor. Add the oats, nut butter, hemp seeds, and matcha powder (if using).

3 Squeeze in the juice of half the lemon and whizz until the mixture is puréed and holds together when squeezed with your fingers. Tip into a bowl and season to taste with salt and pepper and more lemon juice.

4 Divide the mixture into 16 even portions and roll into balls.

5 Heat a large skillet over high heat, add 1½ tablespoons of coconut oil, and cook the balls until lightly golden all over. (You may need to do this in batches, adding more oil to the pan halfway through.)

Alternatives

You can also eat these balls raw. Refrigerate for 1 hour before serving.

Alternatively, bake them on a lightly greased baking tray in the oven at 180°C (160°C fan/350°F/Gas 4) for 20–25 minutes or until lightly golden and heated through.

For one ball: Calories 114 · **Fat** 7.7g · **Carbohydrates** 5.2g · **Sugar** 1.5g
Sodium 33mg · **Fibre** 2g · **Protein** 6.2g · **Cholesterol** 0mg

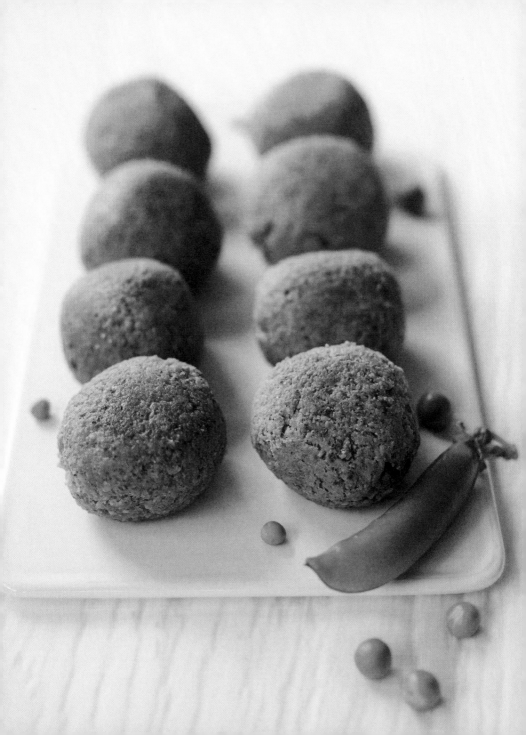

NUT & SEED
NUTRIENT BOOSTERS

*A **HIGH-FIBRE** snack to maintain your energy and **BLOOD SUGAR** levels.*

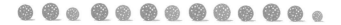

Ingredients

MAKES 16

60g (2oz) chickpeas, soaked overnight (cooked weight about 150g/5½oz)

30g (1oz) brown rice (cooked weight 100g/3½oz)

100g (3½oz) red split lentils (cooked weight 200g/7oz)

75g (2½oz) broccoli, chopped

½ red pepper, deseeded and finely chopped

1 celery stick, finely chopped

25g (1oz) each pumpkin and sunflower seeds

1 tsp thyme leaves

85g (3oz) cashew nuts

50g (1¾oz) whole almonds

½ tsp tamari

1 tsp brown miso paste

sesame or chia seeds, to coat (optional)

Method

1 Drain the soaked chickpeas and rinse under cold water. Place in a pan with 300ml (10fl oz) boiling, salted water. Bring back to the boil, cover, and simmer for 1 hour until the chickpeas are soft, but not soggy – they should have some "bite". Drain and put to one side.

2 Bring the rice to the boil in salted water, then simmer for about 30 minutes until really soft. Drain and put to one side.

3 Rinse the lentils under cold water. Place in a pan with 300ml (10fl oz) boiling, salted water. Bring back to the boil, cover, and simmer for 10 minutes until the lentils are soft, but not soggy. Drain and put to one side.

4 Combine the rice, lentils, raw broccoli, raw pepper, raw celery, seeds, and thyme in a big bowl.

5 Put the chickpeas, nuts, tamari, and miso in a food processor and whizz until you have a rough paste. (You don't want a purée, so don't overdo it!) Add this mixture to the big bowl, combine well and season.

6 Preheat the oven to 200°C (180°C fan/400°F/Gas 6). Line a large baking tray with parchment paper. Divide the mixture into 16 evenly sized portions and roll into balls. If you wish, roll the balls in sesame seeds and/or chia seeds, to coat them. Place on the baking tray.

7 Bake in the preheated oven for 20 minutes until golden brown. Remove and leave to cool on a wire rack for a few minutes before serving hot. Alternatively, serve cold.

For one ball: Calories 111 · **Fat** 6.2g · **Carbohydrates** 9.3g · **Sugar** 1.2g
Sodium 26mg · **Fibre** 1.8g · **Protein** 5.1g · **Cholesterol** 0mg

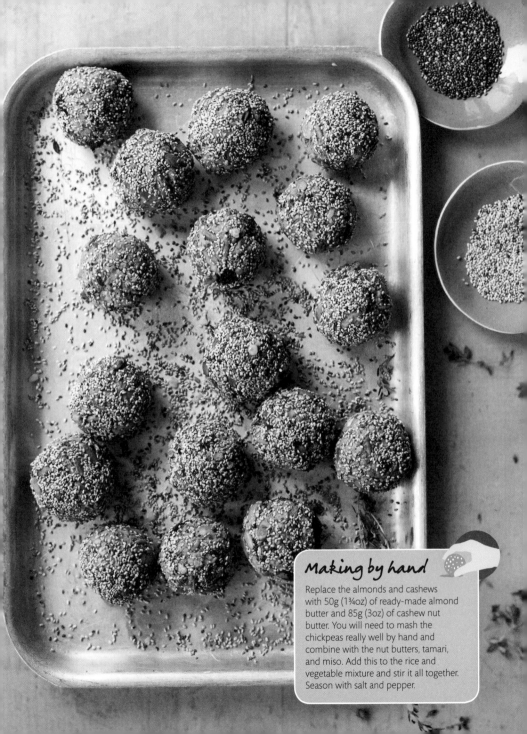

Making by hand

Replace the almonds and cashews with 50g (1¾oz) of ready-made almond butter and 85g (3oz) of cashew nut butter. You will need to mash the chickpeas really well by hand and combine with the nut butters, tamari, and miso. Add this to the rice and vegetable mixture and stir it all together. Season with salt and pepper.

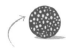

HEMP-COATED
QUINOA CRUNCHERS

Contains FIVE of the top SUPERFOODS for health and vitality.

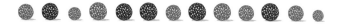

Ingredients

MAKES 16

200g (7oz) raw beetroots

juice of 1 lemon

75g (2½oz) quinoa

300ml (10fl oz) vegetable stock

½–1 red chilli, deseeded and finely chopped

1 garlic clove, crushed

1 tbsp chopped parsley

50g (1¾oz) pecans, chopped

2 tsp ground cumin

pinch of smoked paprika

50g (1¾oz) gram flour

75g (2½oz) shelled hemp seeds

2–3 tbsp coconut oil, if frying

Method

1 Preheat the oven to 180°C (160°C fan/350°F/Gas 4). Place the beetroots, whole, in a baking dish. Cover with foil and bake for about an hour or until very tender when pierced with a small, sharp knife.

2 When cool enough to handle, peel the beetroots, cut into chunks, and whizz in a food processor or mash well with half the lemon juice until puréed. Scrape the purée into a large bowl.

3 Rinse the quinoa in a sieve under cold water, then drain. Bring the stock to the boil in a pan, and tip in the quinoa. Bring back to the boil. Cover, reduce the heat, and simmer for about 20 minutes or until the quinoa is tender and almost all the liquid has been absorbed. Tip into a sieve to drain and cool.

4 Scrape the cooled quinoa into the bowl of puréed beetroot. Add the chilli, garlic, and parsley, then stir in the pecans, cumin, smoked paprika, and flour. Season to taste with salt, pepper, and lemon juice.

5 Shape the mixture into 16 evenly sized balls. Tip the hemp seeds onto a large flat surface and roll the balls evenly in them.

6 Heat a large frying pan over a high heat, add about 1½ tablespoons of coconut oil, and fry the balls until lightly golden all over.

Alternative

Bake the balls on a lightly greased baking tray in the oven at 180°C (160°C fan/350°F/Gas 4) for 20–25 minutes.

For one ball: Calories 80 · **Fat** 4.8g · **Carbohydrates** 6.2g · **Sugar** 1.5g
Sodium 32mg · **Fibre** 1g · **Protein** 3.4g · **Cholesterol** 0mg

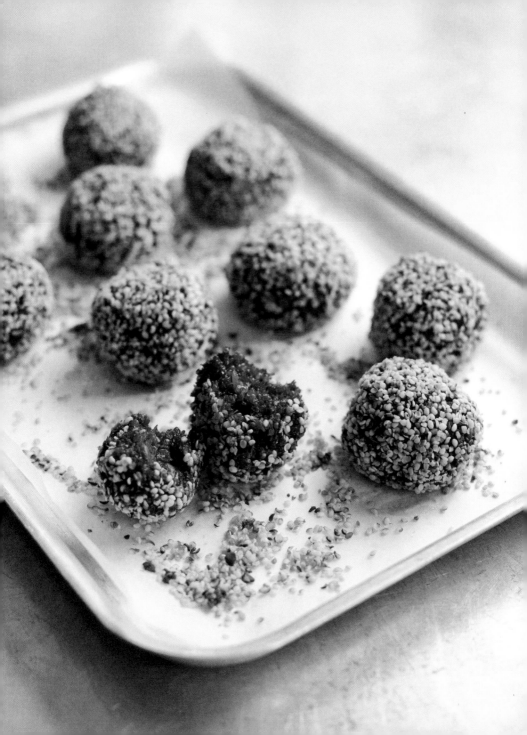

Super STAR NUTS

Cashew

High in magnesium, which is vital for healthy bones, cashews are also rich in iron, phosphorus, zinc, copper, and manganese. They help support memory and concentration.

Pistachio

Packed with 6 grams of protein per ounce, pistachios are little green sticks of dynamite! Full of antioxidants, they also support eye health and regulate hormones.

Brazil

Rich in selenium, a powerful antioxidant, and in minerals that support thyroid function and the immune system, Brazils are also a good source of vitamin E.

Pecan

These nuts can help regulate cholesterol levels and support heart health, as they contain plant sterols and oleic acid, an important monounsaturated fatty acid.

Cashew

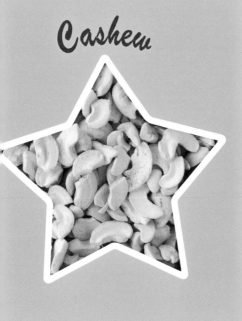

Pistachio

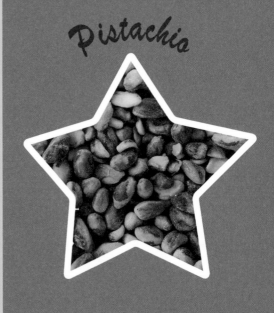

Brazil

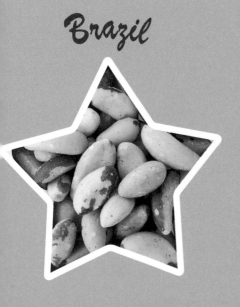

Pecan

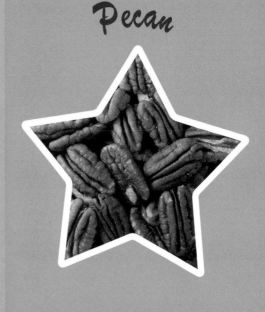

SWEET POTATO
CHILLI BITES

Turmeric, chilli, and cumin help FIRE UP your METABOLISM.

Ingredients

MAKES 16

85g (3oz) dried chickpeas, soaked overnight (cooked weight 200g/7oz)

200g (7oz) sweet potato, unpeeled, chopped

1 tbsp coconut oil

½ red onion, finely chopped

2 garlic cloves, crushed

1 tsp ground turmeric

1 tsp ground cumin

1½ tsp finely chopped red chilli

juice of ½ lemon

2 tbsp tahini

30g (1oz) roughly chopped coriander leaves

Method

1 Drain the soaked chickpeas and rinse under cold water. Place in a pan with 500ml (16fl oz) boiling water, cover, and simmer for around 1 hour until soft.

2 Steam the chunks of sweet potato for 15 minutes until soft.

3 While the sweet potato is steaming, heat the oil in a frying pan and gently fry the onion and garlic until soft. Add the turmeric, cumin, and chilli, and fry for a further 2 minutes.

4 Preheat the oven to 200°C (180°C fan/400°F/Gas 6).

5 Put the chickpeas, sweet potato, lemon juice, tahini, and coriander in a food processor and whizz for about 10 seconds to rough it all up just a little – you definitely don't want to over-blitz it.

6 Tip the contents into a big bowl and add the onion mixture. Season with salt and pepper. Stir well.

7 Divide the mixture into 16 evenly sized portions and roll into balls with your hands. Place them on a baking tray lined with parchment paper and bake in the preheated oven for 20 minutes.

8 Remove and leave to cool on a wire rack for a few minutes to harden up before serving hot. Alternatively, serve cold.

For one ball: Calories 60 · Fat 3.3g · Carbohydrates 5.9g · Sugar 1.3g
Sodium 9mg · Fibre 1.7g · Protein 2.2g · Cholesterol 0mg

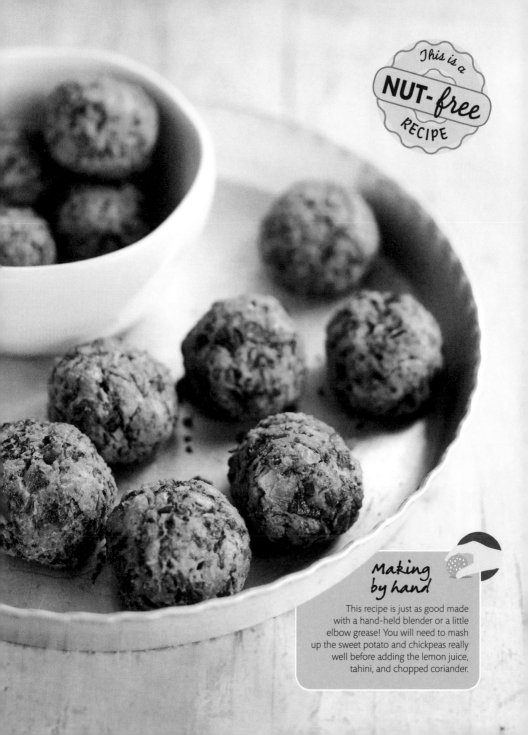

This is a
NUT-free
RECIPE

Making by hand

This recipe is just as good made with a hand-held blender or a little elbow grease! You will need to mash up the sweet potato and chickpeas really well before adding the lemon juice, tahini, and chopped coriander.

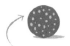

BROCCOLI & MACA
POWERHOUSE BALLS

Packed with C and B vitamins to BOOST YOUR IMMUNITY and energy.

Ingredients

MAKES 16

50g (1¾oz) sunflower seeds

100g (3½oz) hazelnuts

200g (7oz) broccoli, chopped

½ small onion (about 25g/ scant 1oz), finely chopped

2 garlic cloves, crushed

3 tbsp coconut oil, plus extra if frying

2 tbsp tahini

1 tbsp maca powder

¼ tsp ground nutmeg

Method

1 Tip the sunflower seeds into the bowl of a food processor and whizz until they resemble breadcrumbs. Add the remaining ingredients and whizz until the mixture has a paste-like consistency.

2 Tip the mixture into a bowl and season to taste.

3 Divide into 16 evenly sized pieces and roll into balls. Refrigerate for 1 hour before eating raw.

Alternatives

You can also eat these balls hot. Heat a large frying pan over a high heat, add about 1½ tablespoons of coconut oil and fry the balls until lightly golden all over. (You may need to do this in batches, adding more oil to the pan halfway through.)

Alternatively, bake them on a lightly greased baking tray in a preheated oven at 180°C (160° fan/350°F/Gas 4) for 20–25 minutes or until lightly golden and heated through.

For one ball: Calories 107 · Fat 9.8g · Carbohydrates 2g · Sugar 1g
Sodium 3mg · Fibre 1.9g · Protein 2.9g · Cholesterol 0mg

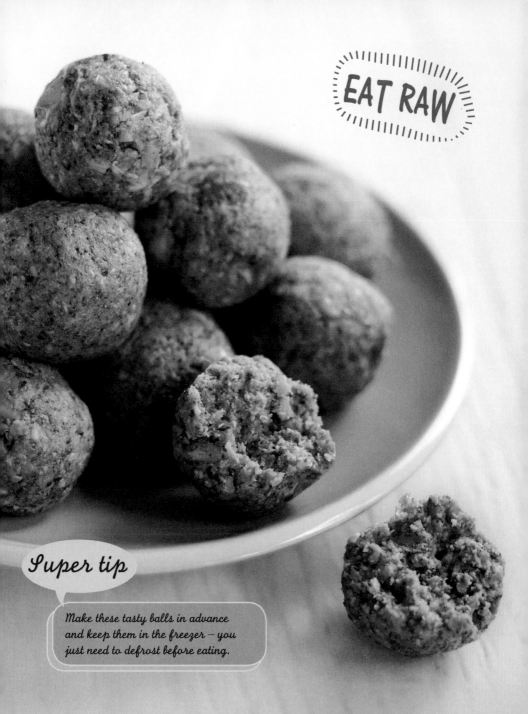

EAT RAW

Super tip

Make these tasty balls in advance
and keep them in the freezer — you
just need to defrost before eating.

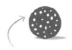

KALE-COVERED
COCONUT BLASTS

*Full of **PROTEIN-RICH EGG** to keep you full for longer.*

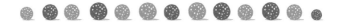

Ingredients

MAKES 18

1 tbsp coconut oil

½ onion, finely chopped

½–1 green chilli, deseeded and finely chopped

½ tsp ground turmeric

1½ tsp garam masala

pinch of ground cinnamon

pinch of ground cloves

400ml (14fl oz) coconut milk

50g (1¾oz) unsweetened desiccated coconut

100g (3½oz) dried green lentils

juice of 1–2 limes, to taste

3 hard-boiled eggs, chopped

2 tbsp chopped coriander

FOR THE COATING

4 tbsp buckwheat flour

2 eggs

large handful of trimmed kale, very finely shredded

50g (1¾oz) pumpkin seeds, chopped

Method

1 Heat the coconut oil in a small pan, add the chopped onion and chilli, and fry gently for about 5 minutes, without browning. Add the spices and fry for a couple of minutes more.

2 Stir in the coconut milk and desiccated coconut, and bring to the boil. Stir in the lentils, reduce the heat, and simmer for 20–25 minutes or until the lentils are very tender and the liquid has thickened. Stir occasionally.

3 Remove from the heat and leave until warm. Tip the mixture into the bowl of a food processor and whizz until you have a coarse paste. Scrape the mixture into a bowl, season according to taste with salt, pepper, and lime juice. Fold in the chopped hard-boiled eggs and coriander.

4 Shape the mixture into 18 evenly sized balls and set aside.

5 Tip the flour onto a plate and season with salt and pepper. Lightly beat the eggs in a bowl. Mix the shredded kale and pumpkin seeds together on a large tray.

6 Roll each ball evenly in the flour, then the egg, shaking off any excess, and finally coat evenly in the kale and pumpkin seeds.

7 Shallow-fry the balls, in batches if necessary, until lightly golden all over and heated through. Be careful as you add the balls to the hot oil, as the kale will make it splutter a little. Serve with lime wedges, if desired.

For one ball: Calories 88 · **Fat** 5g · **Carbohydrates** 7g · **Sugar** 1.7g
Sodium 48mg · **Fibre** 1.7g · **Protein** 4.5g · **Cholesterol** 53mg

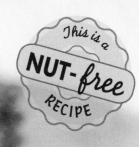

This is a
NUT-free
RECIPE

Lime *wedges*
TO SERVE
(optional)

Fibre-filled FRUIT

Figs

Sweet and crunchy, figs are an excellent source of readily available energy and promote healthy digestion. They are also rich in minerals, including calcium, which supports bone health, and contain high levels of vitamins A, E, and K that contribute to general wellbeing.

Cranberries

These bright red berries are particularly well known for helping the urinary system, keeping infections at bay. They also provide a quick energy boost and are rich in anti-inflammatories.

Dates

As well as tasting deliciously sweet and creamy, dates fortify the immune system and regulate circulation, with their high levels of iron and copper supporting the production of red blood cells. Their slowly released sugars keep energy levels steady.

Apricots

Sweet and sticky, dried apricots boost energy levels. They contain three times more potassium than bananas, helping to protect against high blood pressure and promoting a healthy heart.

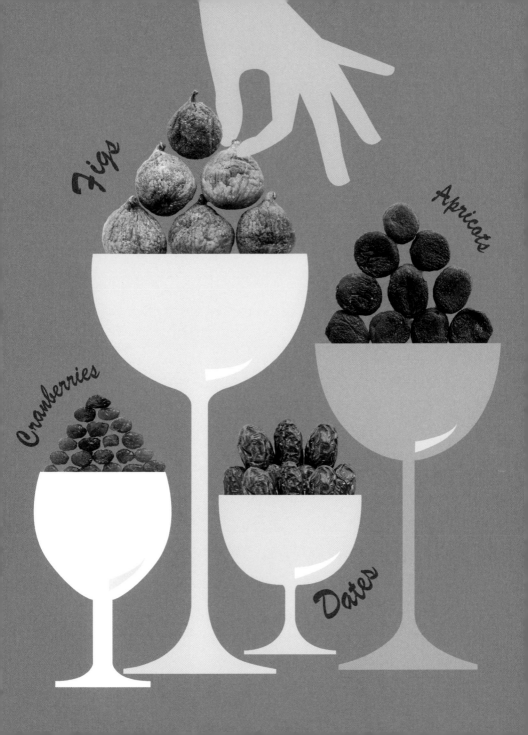

TROPICAL
IMMUNE BOOSTERS

Anti-inflammatory TURMERIC can help protect against colds and flu.

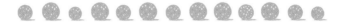

Ingredients

MAKES 16

140g (5oz) dried mango

30g (1oz) goji berries

140g (5oz) cashew nuts

60g (2oz) desiccated coconut, plus extra to coat

1 tbsp baobab powder

1¼ tsp ground turmeric

1 tsp rosehip powder

1 lime, juice and zest

2-4 tbsp cold filtered water

Method

1 Place all the ingredients except the filtered water in a food processor and pulse until finely chopped.

2 With the motor running, add the water a little at a time until the mixture starts to come together, forming a loose ball.

3 Divide into 16 evenly sized portions and roll into balls.

4 Sprinkle a layer of desiccated coconut on a separate plate and gently roll the balls to coat.

5 Place in the fridge for 1 hour or freeze for 20 minutes to firm up before eating. Best served chilled, but absolutely fine to pop in a lunchbox and eat later in the day!

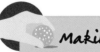

Making by hand

Finely chop the mango (soak your mango in cold water for 5 minutes to soften if necessary), substitute ready-made cashew nut butter for the cashews, and mix in the powders and juice.

For one ball: Calories 92 · **Fat** 4.6g · **Carbohydrates** 11g · **Sugar** 10.5g
Sodium 6mg · **Fibre** 1.2g · **Protein** 2g · **Cholesterol** 0mg

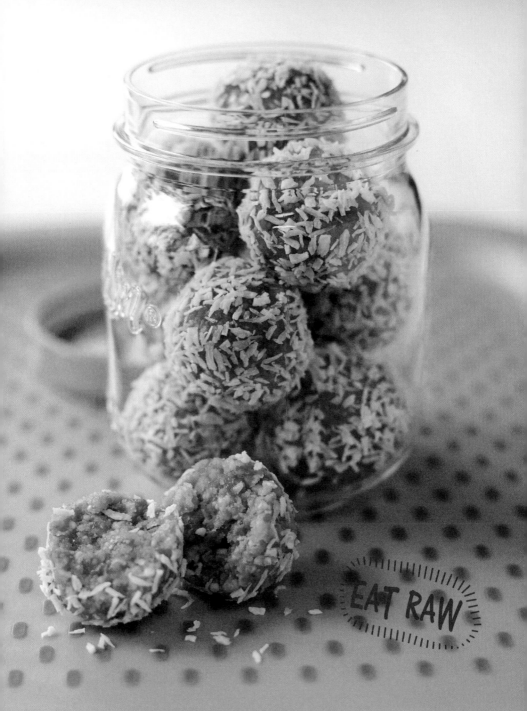

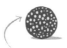

PEANUT BUTTER
& BANANA BALLS

*Includes **MORINGA POWDER** – a nutrient-dense leaf with a spinachy taste.*

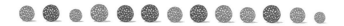

Ingredients

MAKES 16

140g (5oz) crunchy peanut butter, unsalted

1 small ripe banana (about 75g/2½oz)

140g (5oz) dates

30g (1oz) ground flaxseeds

30g (1oz) chia seeds

20g (¾oz) ground almonds

2 tsp moringa powder, to taste

shelled hemp seeds, to coat

Method

1 Place all the ingredients in a food processor and pulse until the mixture starts to come together, forming a loose ball.

2 Divide into 16 evenly sized portions and roll into balls.

3 Sprinkle a layer of hemp seeds on a separate plate and gently roll the balls to coat.

4 Place in the fridge for 1 hour or in the freezer for 20 minutes to firm up before eating. Best served chilled.

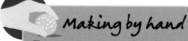

Making by hand

These are very easy to make without a food processor. Simply mash the banana with a fork, finely chop the dates and combine all the ingredients in a large bowl.

For one ball: Calories 92 · **Fat** 4.6g · **Carbohydrates** 11g · **Sugar** 10.5g
Sodium 6mg · **Fibre** 1.2g · **Protein** 2g · **Cholesterol** 0mg

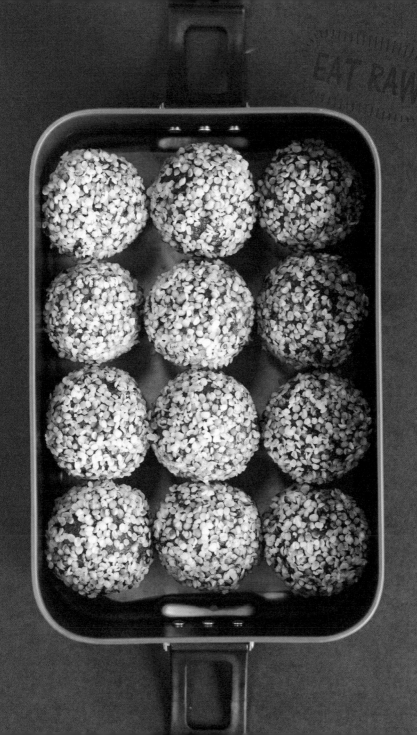

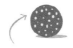

APPLE "PIE"
ANTIOXIDANT BITES

Includes LUCUMA powder for sweetness with a LOW GLYCEMIC index.

Ingredients

MAKES 16

175g (6oz) dried apples

85g (3oz) pecans

50g (1¾oz) rolled oats

2 tbsp maple syrup, or raw honey

1 tbsp lucuma powder

1 tsp ground cinnamon

½ tsp ground nutmeg

¼ tsp ground cloves

2–4 tbsp cold filtered water

raspberry powder, to coat (optional)

Method

1 Place all the ingredients except the filtered water in a food processor and whizz until finely chopped.

2 With the motor running, add the water a little at a time until the mixture starts to come together, forming a loose ball.

3 Divide into 16 evenly sized portions and roll into balls.

4 Sprinkle a layer of raspberry powder on a separate plate and gently roll the balls to coat, if desired.

5 Place in the fridge for 1 hour or in the freezer for 20 minutes to firm up before eating. Best served chilled.

For one ball: Calories 92 · **Fat** 4.6g · **Carbohydrates** 11g · **Sugar** 10.5g
Sodium 6mg · **Fibre** 1.2g · **Protein** 2g · **Cholesterol** 0mg

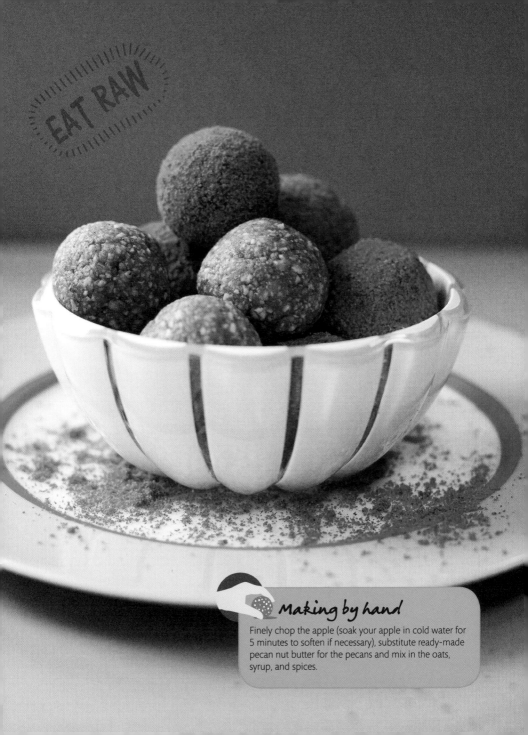

EAT RAW

Making by hand

Finely chop the apple (soak your apple in cold water for 5 minutes to soften if necessary), substitute ready-made pecan nut butter for the pecans and mix in the oats, syrup, and spices.

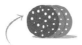

FRUIT & NUT
BUILD-A-BALLS

Coated in **NUTRITIOUS TOPPINGS,** *these make a healthy sweet snack.*

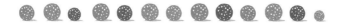

Ingredients

MAKES 16

125g (4½oz) raisins

125g (4½oz) dates, or unsulphured dried apricots

125g (4½oz) walnuts

1–2 tsp spirulina powder, to taste

shelled hemp seeds, cacao powder, unsweetened desiccated coconut, strawberry powder, and crushed pistachio nuts, to coat (optional)

Method

1 Put all the ingredients in a food processor and whizz until combined.

2 Divide the mixture into 16 evenly sized portions and roll into balls with your hands.

3 On separate plates, sprinkle a layer of each of the coatings. Gently roll each ball into one of the coatings.

4 Put the balls in the fridge to firm up for 1 hour before eating. Best served chilled.

Making by hand

Use 125g (4½oz) of ready-made walnut butter instead of walnuts, and chop/mash your choice of dried fruit as super-fine as possible. Put all the ingredients in a bowl, mix, roll, and coat, and hey presto, a more textured build-a-ball!

For one ball: Calories 86 · **Fat** 5.4g · **Carbohydrates** 8.2g · **Sugar** 8.1g
Sodium 8mg · **Fibre** 0.9g · **Protein** 1.8g · **Cholesterol** 0mg

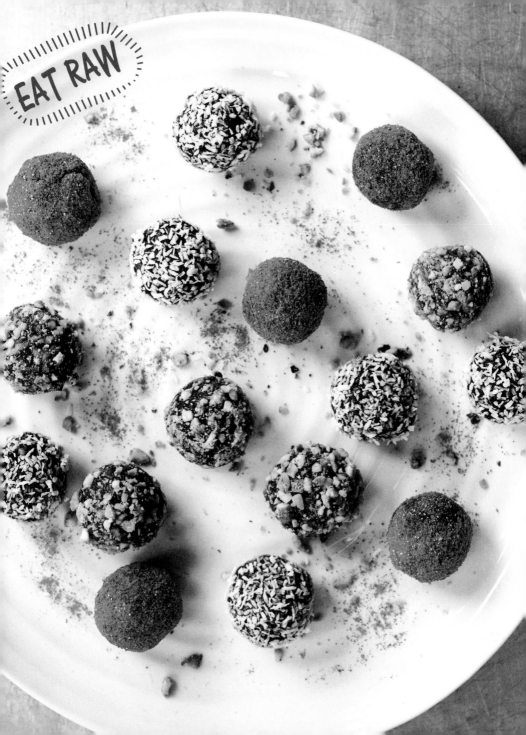

EAT RAW

POWDERS that PACK a PUNCH

Maca

A root that belongs to the radish family, maca was used by Inca warriors to increase strength and stamina before battle. It also regulates hormones and is great for the skin.

Matcha

The finely ground powder of green tea, matcha is high in antioxidants, fortifies the immune system, increases energy, boosts memory and concentration, and detoxes the body.

Acai

The powder of the acai berry has ten times more antioxidants than grapes and in addition to its ability to fight free radicals (that cause cellular breakdown and ageing), it boosts energy and promotes healthy digestion.

Baobab

Derived from the African fruit, this fatigue-fighting powder has six times more vitamin C than oranges, six times more potassium than bananas, and twice as much calcium as milk.

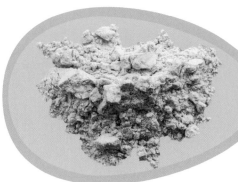

Maca

Matcha

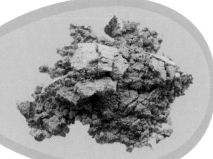

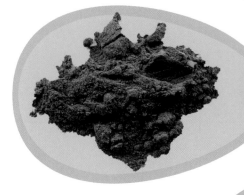

Acai

Baobab

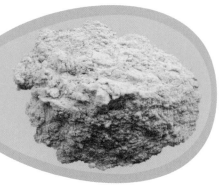

SUPERFOOD
GRANOLA BALLS

*contains **AMINO ACIDS** which help **MUSCLES** recover and repair.*

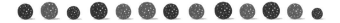

Ingredients

MAKES 16

100g (3½oz) blueberries, fresh or frozen

50g (1¾oz) maple syrup, rice syrup, or raw honey

50g (1¾oz) coconut oil

100g (3½oz) rolled oats

25g (1oz) pumpkin seeds

25g (1oz) sunflower seeds

25g (1oz) chia seeds

50g (1¾oz) flaked almonds

25g (1oz) ground almonds

25g (1oz) raisins

25g (1oz) goji berries

1 tsp ground cinnamon

1–2 tsp acai powder or baobab powder

Method

1 Put the blueberries in a pan with 1 tablespoon of water. Bring to the boil and simmer until the blueberries are really soft and squishy. Add the maple syrup and coconut oil and heat through until combined.

2 Combine all the other ingredients in a big bowl. Add the blueberry mixture to the dry mixture and stir until well combined. The mixture will be sticky. Divide into 16 evenly sized portions and roll into balls.

3 Refrigerate for 1 hour before eating raw.

Alternative

You can also bake these bites. Preheat the oven to 180°C (160°C fan/350°F/Gas 4). Place on a large baking tray lined with parchment paper, and bake for about 15 minutes. Allow to cool and serve.

> **66 GREAT for pre & post WORKOUT ! 99**

For one ball: Calories 125 · **Fat** 8.5g · **Carbohydrates** 9.8g · **Sugar** 4.7g
Sodium 3mg · **Fibre** 1.9g · **Protein** 2.9g · **Cholesterol** 0mg

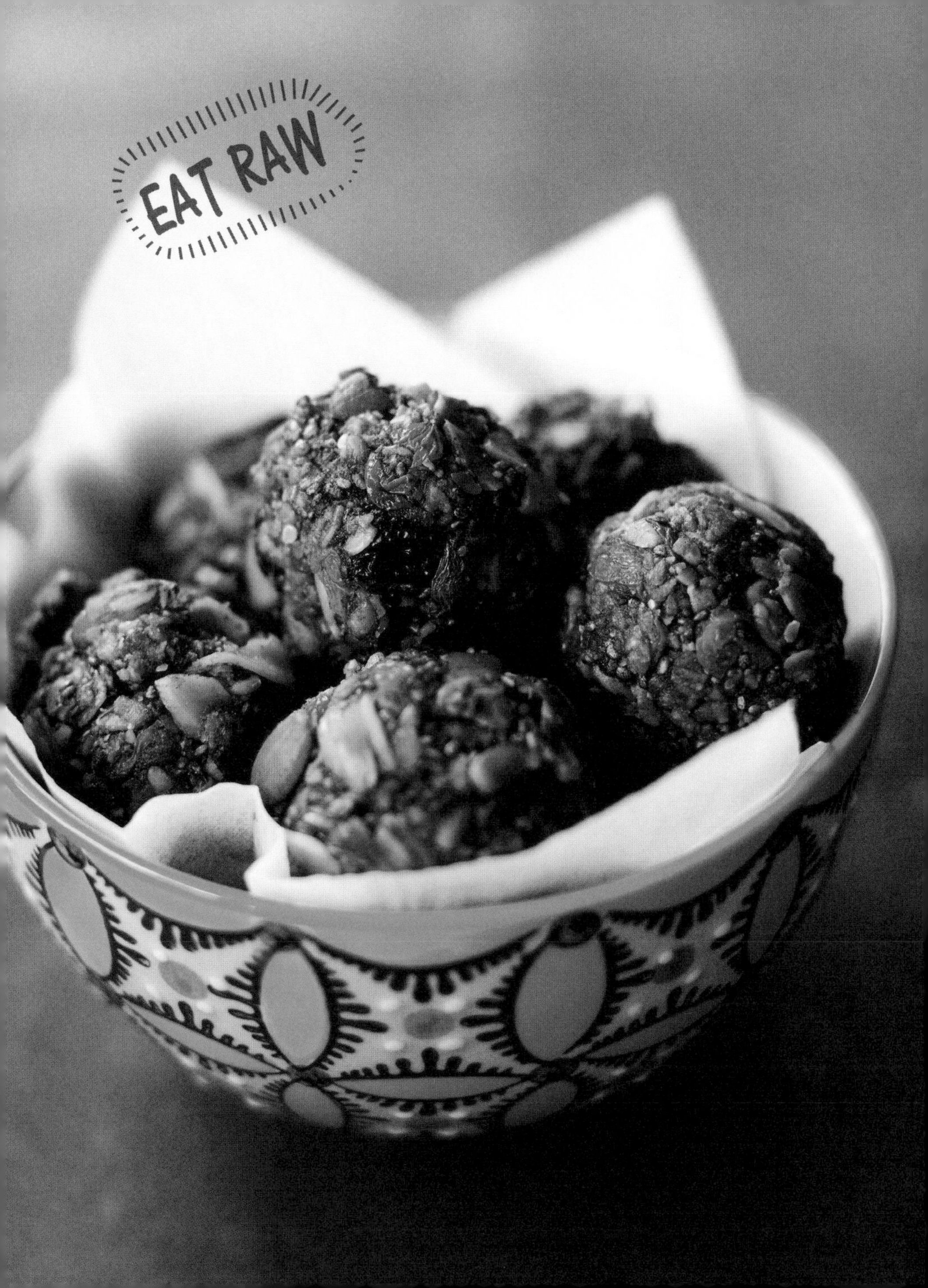
EAT RAW

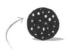

CRANBERRY & FIG
SPICE BITES

The B VITAMINS and ZINC in the MACA POWDER help to maintain stamina.

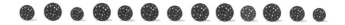

Ingredients

MAKES 16

125g (4½oz) whole almonds

125g (4½oz) dried cranberries (sugar-free)

125g (4½oz) dried figs, stalks removed

1 tsp maca powder

½ tsp ground cinnamon

¼ tsp ground ginger

¼ tsp allspice

¼ tsp ground nutmeg

1½ tbsp orange juice

Method

1 Put all the ingredients in a food processor and blend for about 30 seconds until the mixture is finely chopped.

2 Divide the mixture into 16 evenly sized portions and then roll into balls – you may find this easier to do if your hands are wet.

3 Put the balls in the fridge for 1 hour before eating.

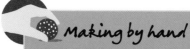

Making by hand

Although these are best made in a food processor, you could also make them by hand. Replace the whole almonds with 125g (4½oz) of ready-made almond butter, chop/mash the dried fruit as finely as possible, and mix in the spices and juice. It's as simple as that!

For one ball: Calories 92 · Fat 4.6g · Carbohydrates 11g · Sugar 10.5g
Sodium 6mg · Fibre 1.2g · Protein 2g · Cholesterol 0mg

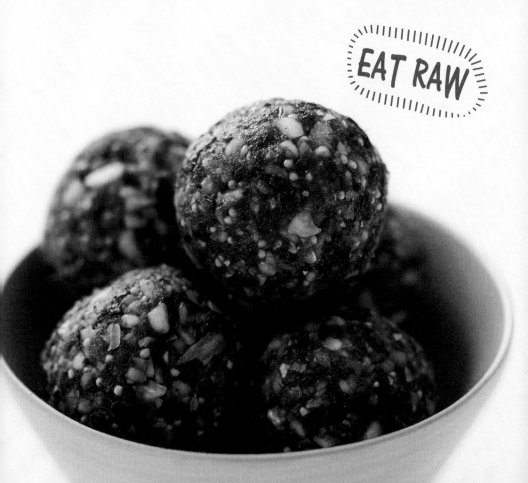

EAT RAW

Super tip

These bites are best with a little bit of texture and "bite", so don't overdo it when you're blending the ingredients in the food processor. You don't want the mixture to be too soft!

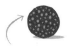

RAW CHOCOLATE
INSTANT ENERGY TREATS

RAW HONEY delivers GUILT-FREE sweetness, while bee pollen is a natural ENERGIZER.

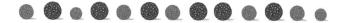

Ingredients

MAKES 16

125g (4½oz) dark tahini

115g (4oz) raw honey, maple syrup, or rice syrup

50g (1¾oz) raw cacao powder

25g (1oz) coconut oil

25g (1oz) ripe avocado

1 tbsp sesame seeds

extra cacao powder, to coat (optional)

bee pollen granules, to coat (optional)

Method

1 Put all the ingredients, except the sesame seeds, in a food processor and whizz until you have a sticky paste. Add the sesame seeds and pulse a few times to combine – the seeds need to remain whole.

2 Refrigerate the mixture for 1 hour so that it firms up a little.

3 Divide the mixture into 16 evenly sized portions and roll into balls. If the mixture is too sticky, wet your hands a little.

4 On separate plates, sprinkle a layer of bee pollen granules and some cacao powder, if desired. Gently roll the balls in one or the other. They should be less sticky now and easy to roll into the perfect shape.

5 Put the balls back in the fridge for at least another hour before eating. Serve chilled.

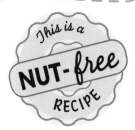

This is a NUT-free RECIPE

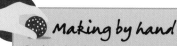

Making by hand

Combine the tahini, honey, cacao powder, and coconut oil (softened) in a small bowl and beat to make a fudgy paste. Put the avocado in a separate bowl and mash to a lump-free consistency (a pestle and mortar works really well here). Add the avocado and sesame seeds to the chocolate mixture and stir them through until combined.

For one ball: Calories 89 · **Fat** 7g · **Carbohydrates** 5g · **Sugar** 4.4g
Sodium 2mg · **Fibre** 1g · **Protein** 1.7g · **Cholesterol** 0mg

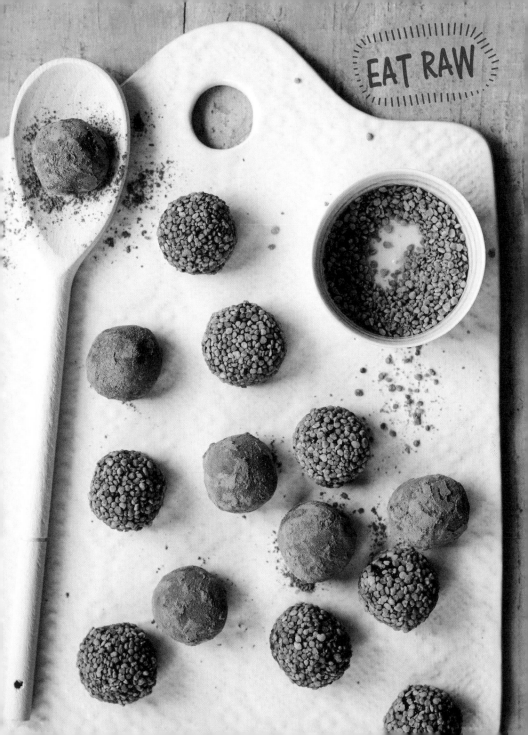

EAT RAW

AVOCADO & BANANA
RECOVERY ICE BITES

with nutrient-loaded chia seeds to **RESTORE ENERGY** *after exercising.*

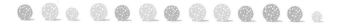

Ingredients

MAKES 8

**8 60-ML (2FL-OZ) SPHERICAL
ICE LOLLY MOULDS OR 16
LARGE ICE-CUBE MOULDS**

400 ml (14fl oz)
unsweetened almond
or hazelnut milk

2 tbsp cacao nibs

1 tbsp chia seeds

½ ripe avocado

1 small banana

pinch of sea salt

Method

1 Pour the almond or hazelnut milk into a small pan and sprinkle in the cacao nibs. Warm gently, bring to a simmer, then remove from the heat. Leave to cool slightly, stir in the chia seeds, then leave to cool completely.

2 Tip the avocado and banana into the bowl of a food processor and blend well with a pinch of salt. Add the cooled milk mixture to the bowl and whizz again, to break up the cacao nibs a little but not so that they are smooth.

3 Using a small plastic funnel or a funnel made from parchment paper, pour the mixture into small spherical moulds. Alternatively, try ice-lolly moulds or large ice-cube trays. Place in the freezer.

4 When the bites are half-frozen, insert a lolly stick or cake pop stick into each one. Return to the freezer and freeze until hard.

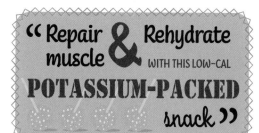

" Repair & Rehydrate muscle WITH THIS LOW-CAL **POTASSIUM-PACKED** *snack "*

For one ball: Calories 23 · **Fat** 1.6g · **Carbohydrates** 2g · **Sugar** 1.1g
Sodium 24mg · **Fibre** 1g · **Protein** 0.5g · **Cholesterol** 0mg

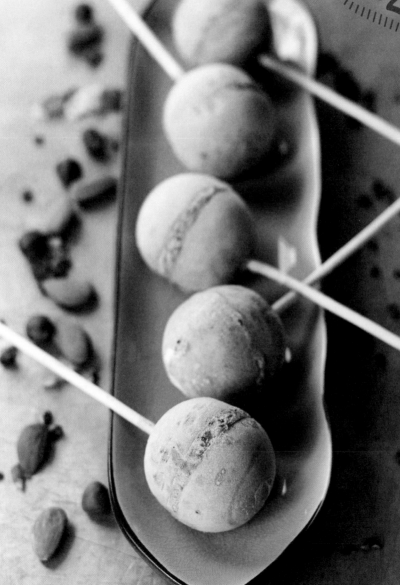

GLOSSARY

Amino acids Used in every cell of the body, amino acids are the building blocks for protein and also aid tissue growth and repair.

Anti-inflammatory Foods with anti-inflammatory properties reduce inflammation in the body and can help fight disease.

Antioxidants These help to neutralize free radicals from the environment, which can damage cells in the body and cause premature ageing.

B vitamins The B vitamin family is made up of eight vitamins. They help the body unlock and use the energy in food, and help to form red blood cells.

Calcium Essential for bone and teeth formation and strength, calcium also regulates nerve and muscle function, hormones, and blood pressure.

Copper Helps the body produce the enzymes it needs for iron absorption, helps to form red blood cells, and maintains skin, bone, and nerve formation.

Fibre Can help prevent heart disease, diabetes, weight gain, and some cancers, and can also improve digestive health.

Folate (vitamin B9) Also referred to as folic acid, folate promotes a healthy nervous system, and is particularly important for pregnant women to ensure babies develop properly in the womb.

Free radicals Unstable and highly reactive molecules that exist in the environment around us and are said to cause damage to cells, accelerating the ageing process.

Glycemic index A number that indicates a food's effect on blood glucose (also called blood sugar) levels. Foods with a lower glycemic index will have less of an effect on blood sugar, whereas foods with a high glycemic index may cause blood sugar to become unstable.

HDL cholesterol High density lipoprotein, also referred to as "good" cholesterol, carries excess cholesterol back to the liver for processing. High HDL levels in the blood reduce the risk of heart disease.

Iron Important for red blood cell function, energy release, and growth. A lack of iron in the blood causes anaemia.

Lauric acid Found in coconuts, this is converted in the body into a highly beneficial compound called monolaurin, which has antiviral and antibacterial properties.

Magnesium Important for DNA repair, energy production, heart, and circulation health.

Manganese An antioxidant mineral that is important in bone and ligament formation.

Metabolism The rate at which your body burns energy – or calories – to fuel everyday cell processes and growth.

Monounsaturated fatty acids Improves blood cholesterol levels, which can decrease the risk of heart disease. May also benefit insulin levels and help to control blood sugar.

Omega-3 These essential fatty acids regulate inflammation, promote healthy brain function, and are vital for healthy skin, eyes, and joints.

Phosphorus Important for healthy bones, phosphorus also supports energy production and activates B vitamins in the body.

Phyto-nutrients These plant-based compounds have beneficial effects on the body, working with other essential nutrients to promote good health.

Phytosterols Plant compounds called phytosterols are structurally similar to cholesterol, and can act in the intestine to lower cholesterol absorption and therefore reduce the risk of heart disease.

Potassium Vital for blood pressure regulation, potassium also regulates the balance of hormones in the body and promotes nerve and muscle health.

Selenium An antioxidant mineral that can fight cancer-causing compounds and is important for reproductive health and fertility.

Vitamin A Also known as retinol, this is important for eye health and vision and for collagen production, which keeps skin healthy. It helps the immune system fight infection.

Vitamin C Supports the immune system and promotes healthy bones, teeth, and gums. Also important in the absorption of iron by the body.

Vitamin E This antioxidant vitamin supports the skin, heart, and circulation, and is important for healthy growth.

Vitamin K Found in green, leafy vegetables, this helps to regulate the blood-sugar balance in the body, heals wounds, and also supports a healthy heart and circulatory system.

Zinc An important mineral that regulates the immune system, aids healing, and supports healthy skin, hair, and muscles.

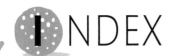

INDEX

The Authors

Kate Turner has been creating deliciously healthy, happy food for herself and her family for decades. She loves good, honest, tasty meals that make you feel amazing, are packed full of natural energy, and are super quick and easy to prepare! Kate shares her ideas about food, foraging, gardening, and family life on Instagram and her blog Homegrown Kate (homegrownkate. com). Thanks go to her children, Stan, Scarlet, and Tommy, for being the best taste-testing team!

Annie Nichols contributed the recipes on pages 26-7, 30-1, 36-9, and 58-9. Originally a trained chef, Annie is a well-established cookery writer, food columnist, photographer, and food stylist. She can be contacted at www. hotmealsnow.com.

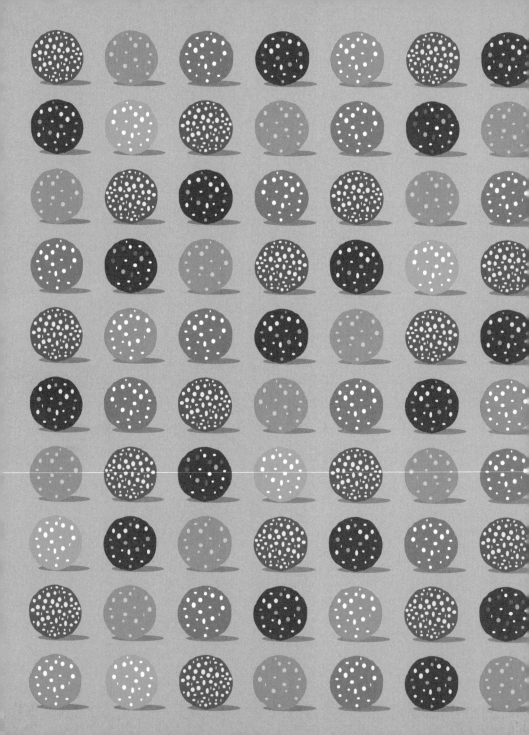